Smoothies!
Become a Smoothie Alchemist

Kimberly Wechsler

Smoothies!

Become a Smoothie Alchemist © 2014 Kimberly Wechsler

Proudly Published by Fitness Productions, LLC

All rights reserved. No portion of this book may be reproduced mechanically, electronically, or by any other means, including photocopying, without written permission of the publisher. It is illegal to copy this book, post it to a website, or distribute it by any other means without permission form the publisher.

Kimberly Wechsler

www.FitAmericanFamilies

Phone: (972) 672-6276

Disclaimer: This publication contains opinions and ideas of its author and her experiences teaching nutrition, wellness and exercises to families. It is intended to provide helpful and informative material on the subject matter covered. It is sold with the understanding that the author and publisher are not engaged in rendering professional services in this book. If the reader requires personal assistance or professional advice, a competent professional should be consulted.

The author and publisher specifically disclaim any responsibility for any liability, loss or risk, personal or otherwise, which is incurred as a consequence, directly or indirectly, by the use and application of any contents of this book.

Smoothies! Become a Smoothie Alchemist

ISBN 978-0-9889464-8-4

About the Author

Kimberly Wechsler, CHHC, AADP, CPT, is a popular and recognizable Family Fitness Specialist, Nutritionist, Health Activist and Author. She is a 22- year fitness industry leader specializing in fitness, nutrition and healthy lifestyles. She has taught over 75,000 children and families how to live more healthfully.

For more information about Kimberly go to;
www.FitAmericanFamilies.com

Kimberly's other Books:

101 Cool Pool Games, Hunter House Publishing I.S.B.N.978-0-89793-483-1

101 Juegos De Piscina Para Niño's I.S.B.N. 978-84-95973-52-8

303 Preschooler-Approved Active Games and Exercises, Hunter House Publishing I.S.B.N.978-0-89793-618-7

303 Kid-Approved Active Games and Exercises, Hunter House Publishing I.S.B.N.978-0-89793-619-4

303 'Tween-Approved Active Games and Exercises, Hunter House Publishing I.S.B.N.978-0-89793-620-0

Why Should I Drink Water? Fitness Productions, LLC, I.S.B.N.978-0-9889464-3-9

Family Games, Fitness Productions, LLC. I.S.B.N.978-0-9889464-4-6

Boot Camp Fitness for Kids, Fitness Productions, LLC I.S.B.N. 978-0-9889464-5-3

Smoothies! Become a Smoothie Alchemist

To my beautiful children Andrew and Addison.

You have made me stronger, better

and more fulfilled than I could have ever imagined.

Smoothies! Become a Smoothie Alchemist

Table of Contents

Introduction 6

Become a Smoothie Alchemist 8

10 Gift from the Elixir of Living Foods 15

Not All Smoothies Are Created Equal 18

The Masterwork 20

The Alchemy of Smoothies 24

Smoothie Science 39

Smoothie Troubleshooting 42

The Formula's 44

Red/Orange Smoothies 44

Yellow/Beige Smoothies 61

Green Smoothies 70

Blue/Purple Smoothies 82

Brown Smoothies 94

Introduction

"And, when you want something, all the universe conspires in helping you to achieve it."

—Paulo Coelho, The Alchemist

We all have one desire in common, and that is to live healthier lives. One important factor in living a healthy lifestyle is based upon the foods we eat. The food we eat gives our bodies the information and materials it needs to function properly. If we don't get the right information, our metabolic processes suffer and our health declines. By choosing the "right foods" we increase the chances of living a healthier life and reduce our chances of diseases such as heart disease, stroke, cancer and diabetes.

So what type of diet is best for disease prevention and to maintain a healthy weight? The answer may surprise you, the best diet is one that you can stick with for life, not a fad diet that is dangerous or difficult to maintain, but a diet that you and your family will enjoy and can easily fit into your lifestyle. Abundant evidence suggests that the most healthful diets include large amounts of vegetables and fruits. Are you eating enough fruit and vegetables daily? We all know that fruits and vegetables can improve our health in a powerful way, but we seem to keep coming up with reasons why we can't eat more of them. I know it can seem difficult to eat a banana, an orange, a handful of berries and a cup of yogurt in one sitting, but there is a way to eat this healthfully, everyday-drink a smoothie!

Smoothies are a blended drink made from fresh fruit vegetables and any other healthy ingredients you wish to add. They have a milkshake like consistency that is thicker than slushy drinks. Smoothies became widely available in the United States in the late 1960s when ice cream vendors and health food stores began to sell them. By the 1990s and 2000s, smoothies became available at mainstream cafés and coffee shops and in pre-bottled versions at supermarkets all over the world. Smoothies can range from low calorie to high calorie drinks; they can cost from pennies a glass to $10 per glass. Do you know where to find the healthiest and the least expensive smoothies? YOUR HOME!

Smoothies began in my kitchen over 20 years ago when my kids barely had time for breakfast; I thought I was doing a pretty good job getting my kids to drink Carnation Instant Breakfast every morning. Until one morning I went to the pantry to get their instant breakfast drink when I realized I didn't have any left. So I pulled out my blender and tried to make my own version of a drinkable breakfast. I added milk, yogurt, chocolate syrup, a banana and ice into a blender; poured it into a glass and my kids said it was the best breakfast drink they ever drank. This was one of those "aha" moments for me. I appreciated how easy smoothies are to make and I can make them as healthy as I want, I am in control, so I decided to play around with the ingredients. As I became confident in my smoothie making skills I realized that I could increase the number of fruits and vegetables my kids consumed each day by adding them to the smoothie. So, I began to experiment with other tastes, textures and supplements and some pretty wacky ingredients, each morning they had a new concoction. This was great, I was feeling pretty proud of myself, I was able to get my kids to "drink" their fruits and vegetables every morning or for an after school snack and I started sneaking in some other foods that my kids would never eat for breakfast-who knew breakfast could be so healthy and so easy? That's the day I became a smoothie alchemist. My kids nicknamed me "The Mad Scientist of Smoothies!" Okay I didn't think The Mad Scientist of Smoothies was a good name for this book, so I nicknamed myself after one of my favorite books, "The Smoothie Alchemist."

Become a Smoothie Alchemist

It is so easy to make smoothies and the possibilities are endless. By blending nutritious foods together you can make it easier to enjoy a larger volume of fruit and vegetables than you would otherwise, increasing the amount of nutrients you put into your body. When you make your own smoothie you can add fresh whole fruits and nuts, grains such as rolled oats and minimize the sugars by adding alternatives such as honey. The extra fiber from the oats and fruits will make you feel full for longer periods which will help you control your appetite. In addition, fiber in your food is known to help slow-down the release of sugar into the blood. This stops a surge of sugar that can trigger hormone release, and results in more stable blood sugar levels and helps control sugar cravings. You also can add other ingredients to create a high protein shake. This ingredients include low fat milk, yogurt, whey extracts from skim milk, wheat germ, protein powder, nuts and other healthy ingredients. But beware you measure these ingredients carefully and add up all the calories in them to keep the smoothie within the calorie cap you have set. You are in control, if there is a certain vitamin or mineral you want to focus on, you can easily modify your smoothie recipe to accommodate your needs. Not only the flavor combinations are infinite, you can prepare different recipes to benefit from specific health components from its ingredients. Using fresh raw fruits and vegetables are considered live foods. These live foods (living foods) contain a wide range of vital life force nutrients, vitamins, minerals, amino acids, oxygen and live enzymes. Their nutritional properties are essential to the proper maintenance of human bodily functions.

Recommended daily serves of fruit and vegetables by age

Age	Fruit	Vegetables
4-7	1-2	2-4
8-11	1-2	3-5
12+	3-4	4-9

Fruits and vegetables are good for your health! They have many vitamins, minerals and other natural substances that help you stay healthy and help your children grow healthy and strong! Here is a brief summary of just some of the vitamins and minerals found in fruits and vegetables.

Calcium: Calcium is essential for healthy bones and teeth. It is also needed for normal functioning of muscles, nerves and some glands.

Fiber: Diets rich in dietary fiber have been shown to have a number of beneficial effects, including decreased risk of coronary heart disease. Drinking fruit smoothies can help you reach the recommended intake of fiber, which is 25 grams for women and 38 grams for men. One serving of fruit typically contains two to four grams of fiber with blackberries, pears and apples having the highest concentration of five to seven grams per serving. The soluble fiber found in fruit helps slow digestion and may help control blood sugar and lower cholesterol.

Folate: Healthful diets with adequate folate may reduce a woman's risk of having a child with a brain or spinal cord defect.

Iron: Needed for healthy blood and normal functioning of all cells.

Magnesium: Magnesium is necessary for healthy bones and is involved with more than 300 enzymes in your body! Inadequate levels may result in muscle cramps and high blood pressure.

Potassium: Diets rich in potassium may help to maintain a healthy blood pressure.

Sodium: Needed for normal cell function throughout the body.

Vitamin A: Keeps eyes and skin healthy and helps protect against infections.

Vitamin C: Helps heal cuts and wounds and keeps teeth and gums healthy.

Smoothies! Become a Smoothie Alchemist

Colorful fruits and vegetables contain disease fighting compounds called phytonutrients. These powerhouses act as super heroes, fighting off free radicals that cause cancer and a host of other enemies that increase your risk of heart disease, diabetes, osteoporosis, and more. The most vibrantly colored fruits and vegetables have the most nutrition, the different antioxidants create the different colors in fruits and veggies so eating an array of colors just ensure that you get the benefits of all of them.

Each different color fruit and vegetables contains unique health components that are essential to our health. Here are just a few of the benefits of color in fruits and vegetables:

Red Fruits and Vegetables

Contain nutrients such as lycopene, ellagic acid, quercetin, and hesperidin, to name a few. These nutrients reduce the risk of prostate cancer, lower blood pressure, reduce tumor growth and LDL cholesterol levels, scavenge harmful free-radicals, and support join tissue in arthritis cases. Lycopene is the predominant pigment in reddish fruits and veggies, is a powerful antioxidant that has been associated with a reduced risk of some cancers, especially prostate cancer, and protection against heart attacks.

Red apples

Blood Oranges

Cherries

Cranberries

Red Grapes

Pink/Red Grapefruit

Red Pears

Pomegranates

Raspberries

Smoothies! Become a Smoothie Alchemist

Strawberries

Watermelon

Beets

Red Peppers

Rhubarb

Tomatoes

Yellow Fruit and Vegetables

Orange/yellow group represent beta-cryptoxanthin and vitamin C also rich in beta-carotene, which are particularly good antioxidants. Helps lowering cholesterol and helps reduce the risk of stroke. These nutrients reduce age-related macular degeneration and the risk of prostate cancer, promote collagen formation and healthy joints, fight harmful free radicals, encourage alkaline balance, and work with magnesium and calcium to build healthy bones.

Apples

Apricots

Bananas

Cape Gooseberries

Cantaloupe *Use by itself or with other melons

Grapefruit

Golden Kiwifruit

Lemons

Mangoes

Nectarines

Oranges

Smoothies! Become a Smoothie Alchemist

Papayas

Yellow Pears

Persimmons

Tangerines

Yellow Watermelon

Carrots

Yellow Peppers

Pumpkin

Butternut Squash

Corn

Yellow White Peaches

Yellow Tomatoes

Green Fruit and Vegetables

The nutrients found in these vegetables reduce cancer risks, lower blood pressure and LDL cholesterol levels, normalize digestion time, support retinal health and vision, fight harmful free-radicals, and boost immune system activity.

These foods exhibit a richness in lutein, particularly beneficial for eye health. Green vegetables contain chlorophyll, fiber, lutein, zeaxanthin, calcium, folate, vitamin C, calcium, and Beta-carotene.

Avocados

Basil

Barley Grass

Bok Choy

Celery

Smoothies! Become a Smoothie Alchemist

- Chard
- Cilantro
- Cucumber
- Endive
- Green apples
- Green Grapes
- Honeydew * Use by itself or with other melons
- Kiwifruit
- Lettuce
- Lemongrass
- Limes
- Green Peas
- Arugula
- Celery
- Kale
- Green Peppers
- Parsley
- Spinach
- Sprouts
- Watercress
- Wheat Grass

Blue/Purple Fruit and Vegetables

Contain nutrients which include lutein, zeaxanthin, resveratrol, vitamin C, fiber, flavonoids, ellagic acid, and quercetin. Similar to the previous nutrients, these nutrients support retinal health, lower LDL cholesterol, boost immune system activity, support healthy digestion, improve calcium and other mineral absorption, fight inflammation, reduce tumor growth, act as an anticarcinogens in the digestive tract, and limit the activity of cancer cells. The purple in grapes helps prevent heart disease.

Blackberries

Blueberries

Black Currants

Concord Grapes

Dates

Dried Plums

Elderberries

Grape Juice (100%)

Purple Figs

Plums

Purple Grapes

Raisins

Purple Carrots

Ten Gifts from the Elixir of Living Foods

#1. Smoothies make it easy to consume your daily intake of fruits and vegetables.

You should aim to consume at least nine servings of vegetables and fruits each day, but consuming so much produce can prove daunting for some. One of the major benefits of smoothies is that they allow you to consume several servings of vegetables and fruits in one sitting. To maximize your vegetable intake without significantly impacting the taste of your smoothies, choose vegetables with a mild flavor, such as spinach, and then add fruit or other mild vegetables to your smoothie.

#2. Smoothies have the Superfood effects

The base of all smoothies in this book are fruits and vegetables. Fruits and vegetables are superfoods. What is a superfood? Food that are a special category of foods found in nature. By definition they are calorie sparse and nutrient dense meaning they pack a lot of punch for their weight as far as goodness goes. They are superior sources of anti-oxidants and essential nutrients - nutrients we need but cannot make ourselves.

#3. Smoothies are quick and easy to make.

Most smoothies take less than 4 minutes to prepare.

#4. Kids like smoothies.

I know that it is difficult to get your kids to eat the recommended amount of fruits and vegetables every day, but it's easy with a smoothie. Find something simple that they'll drink, then slowly over time work in the spinach and other greens. My kids have had a smoothie almost every day of their life, they are both in college now and I am proud to say they have become a Smoothie Alchemist.

#5. Smoothies can be a tasty and easy weight to lose weight.

This applies only if you make healthy smoothies, be sure to read the section of unhealthy ingredients. Many diets promote drinking a meal and making your own smoothie is easy and less expensive than buying store bought smoothies. Vary the type of smoothie you make, one day make a vegetable based smoothie, next day a fruit smoothie, or blend fruits and vegetables together. If you are diabetic, be aware of the fruits with a high sugar content.

#6. Smoothies promote regularity.

One other great thing about smoothies is that it keeps all the natural fiber, which help cleansing the digestive tract. The powerful detox foods that go into it help your liver to detox naturally, and they can help you stay healthy and look great.

#7. Smoothies provide meal flexibility.

Smoothies are a meal. You can easily add protein ingredients (yogurt, milk, whey, eggs) to the smoothie or shake, making it a more balanced, nutritious meal.

They stabilize blood sugar and energy levels. Because smoothies contain fiber, the sugar and calories from smoothies are more slowly absorbed into the blood stream. As a result, your blood sugar levels remain stable and so does your energy. Since smoothies contain fiber, you will feel full longer. High-fiber content means it will take longer to digest, meaning you won't become hungry very quickly. You can consume a smoothie at any meal, not just breakfast. No time for lunch, make a quick smoothie.

#8. Smoothies are inexpensive to make.

The number one excuse for not eating the required five servings of fruits and vegetables each day is they are too expensive. Use fruit that is in season, or buy frozen fruits and vegetables, they retain the majority of their nutritional value and they can be an excellent alternative when certain foods are out of season. Look for fruits that are on sale at your grocery store, if you are not going to eat them or drink them that day, freeze them. Instead of using fruit juice as a smoothie base, opt for filtered water with whole fruit or coconut water. You can add a little sweet with some stevia, which doesn't affect blood sugar and is 100 percent natural.

#9. Become a smoothie alchemist.

Tailor your smoothies to meet your desired health goals. Blending a couple of servings of colorful fruits and vegetables into a smoothie helps ensure you meet your body's daily nutritional needs and you can add any additional supplements superfoods easily into your smoothie.

#10. Smoothies save you money.

Making your own smoothies can help prevent fruit from going to waste, while providing benefits that will keep you on the right track towards good health.

Not All Smoothies Are Created Equal

We all know which ingredients make a smoothie healthy: fruit and veggies. But what about smoothies that contain fruit and/or veggies along with other ingredients. How healthy are they?

Many people think that because it's called a smoothie, it must be healthy. But if you take ingredients that are loaded with sugar, fat, calories and other unhealthy ingredients and stick it in a blender, it's still a bunch of junk. Even if you call it "smoothie." Most restaurants, chains, serving smoothies generally lean towards the unhealthy. One well known Smoothie chain creates a smoothie with 1750 calories in one cup! Know what goes in to your smoothie, before it becomes a sugary slush, and ask how many calories are in your smoothie.

Let's take a look at ingredients to avoid in your smoothies.

Unhealthy Ingredients

Sugar laden fruit juices

Tap water (contaminants)

Ice cream and sherbet

Chemicals

Additives

Chocolate syrups

Flavored syrups

Candy

Sugar

Non-organic peanut butters

Cookies

Pudding mix

Smoothies! Become a Smoothie Alchemist

Cool Whip or whip cream

Soda

Artificial sweetener

Artificial ingredients

The best way to know the exact ingredients in your smoothie is to make them yourself.

The Masterwork

To make a healthy smoothie, start with healthy ingredients.

Fresh is best. The fresher the juice and ingredients you use in your smoothie, the better the flavor and nutrition. Use organic ingredients in your smoothie whenever possible, not only to increase nutrition and avoid pesticides, but also for better taste.

The best vegetables for green smoothies are dark leafy greens as these are the vegetables we struggle to eat the most of and they are the best for us. You can put other vegetables in the blender too but ensure you have enough creamy fruit to balance out the fibrous textures. Fresh raw green leafy vegetables contain high doses of chlorophyll, easily digestible proteins, enzymes and a wide range of vitamins and minerals. These particular vegetables act as mini-transfusions for the blood, a health tonic for the brain and immune system and a cleanser of the kidneys. Try any of the following: rocket, lettuce, parsley, kale, chard, basil, cilantro, bok choy, celery, spinach, dandelion greens, watercress, endive, chicory, broccoli sprouts, mustard sprouts and cucumber are all great in green smoothies. The darker the leaf the better it is for you. You can also add beet tops, celery leaves and strawberry leaves in to your green smoothie. If you are looking for a mild green, the best green to start with is spinach as you can easily hide the taste with sweet fruit.

Fresh herbs. You can include herbs to make the green smoothie taste very fresh. I personally love herbs in my green smoothies. In the summer, toss in some fresh herbs from your garden, a strawberry basil smoothie is fantastic. Other herbs to consider: lemongrass, lavender, and cilantro. Fresh herbs contain antioxidants and are very low in calories.

Canned or jar fruit is good as long as it doesn't have sugar added. Pineapple, applesauce, peaches, plums, and cherries any fruit, even fruit cocktail, unsweetened. Canned apricot nectar lends a uniquely textural sweetness.

Dried is good although soaking your dried fruits and vegetables overnight in water although the blender to incorporate the fruit better in the smoothie. Remember to remove the pits, yep I forgot to remove the pit and it damaged one of my blenders.

Frozen is fine. I have been adding frozen spinach to my green smoothies for years. However on many frozen vegetables there is a warning telling you not to eat them raw. This is because they haven't followed the same safety guidelines as they do for frozen fruit as they expect people to cook their greens and eat their fruit raw. Once the greens are cooked they are much safer to use. Some people reason that if you consume your greens raw, the benefits they provide for your body (and ability of your body to fight off infections) outweighs the risks of eating raw frozen greens. To be safe, please real the package of your frozen food.

Can you freeze greens for green smoothies?

Yes you can freeze any of your greens for use in green smoothies. It will be better to freeze them in portions that you are going to drop straight in your smoothie as you won't easily be able to separate the greens once they are frozen. It is better to chop your greens before freezing them in small portions as your blender won't be able to cope with a large batch of frozen greens. You may even have to defrost our greens for a while before use if your blender isn't very powerful.

Ice vs. frozen fruit

Through my experience, and the number of blenders that I have ruined, I prefer not to use ice in my smoothies; instead I freeze all of my fruits and some of my vegetables ahead of time. When you add ice to your smoothies it will make it more slush like, but it can water down the taste of smoothies as well, another option to pour your smoothie over ice.

If you choose to add ice cubes to your drink, I recommend that you add no more than ½ cup of crushed ice. Crushec ice works breaks up much easier and is easier on your blender better than cubed ice.

HOW TO FREEZE YOUR FRUIT

Freezing fruit is a super easy way to save the great flavors of ripe in-season fruit to enjoy in your smoothies later. If I see fruit beginning to look a little brown, I prepare them immediately for freezing, therefore I never throw any fruit away, ever. Plus when you want to use your frozen fruit, you don't need to thaw the fruit, just put the frozen fruit right into your blender.

1. Prepare the Fruit

All fruit should be rinsed clean and patted dry before freezing.

Apples, pears need to be cored, peeled, and quartered or sliced and then tossed with a bit of lemon juice or cider vinegar to keep them from browning. Grapes –nothing just wash and freeze. Apricots should be halved and pitted. Berries of any type can be left whole. Cherries will be easier to use later if you pit them now. Melons can be cut into cubes or slices or scooped into bite-size balls. Pineapples should be cored and sliced. Stoned fruit such as peaches, plums, and nectarines should be pitted and peeled and may be sliced or cut into wedges. Strawberries need to be hulled and can be cut in half. Banana's just remove the skin.

2. Freeze the Fruit

If you are freezing just one or two pieces of fruit at a time, just follow step one and put them into a freezer zip-lock baggie. Fruit prepared this way will stick together so you will have to use the entire bag at once unless you can break up the pieces carefully. This is my favorite way to freeze fruits, I just put a variety in a zip lock baggie and then I just pop them into the blender straight from the bag. It's a lot cheaper to make individual serving sizes, then to buy them from a store. When preparing a lot of fruit, lay the prepared fruit in a single layer on a large baking sheet or pan (make sure it fits flat in your freezer first!). You can line the pan with parchment paper, waxed paper, or aluminum foil, if you like. Make sure the fruit isn't crowded and is touching as little as possible, otherwise they will stick together. Place in freezer until fruit is frozen solid. This usually takes an hour or two.

3. Transfer Fruit for Frozen Storage

Once fruit is frozen through, transfer it to heavy-duty freezer bags. If you are freezing a variety of fruit, mix and match each bag for making your smoothies.

Frozen fruit will last up to a year in a stand-alone freezer that isn't opened and closed a lot, and up to 6 months in a frequently opened refrigerator-freezer.

4. *Extra Healthy Tip.*
Make coconut water ice cubes instead of tap water ice cubes. This will add nutrients including potassium, magnesium and other electrolytes, and the smoothie flavors will not be greatly changed.

5. *Too much smoothie?*
If you don't have anyone to share your batch of smoothie you can also freeze portion sizes of it in glass containers and thaw out the night before in a bind.

EQUIPMENT:

In the past 15 years of making smoothie I have burned out 5 blenders and damaged the blades of 2 blenders. Now I have a Vitamix and it blends everything, including ice, I highly recommend this blender, I am sure there are other blenders just as good, but this is the blender I have used in the past 8 years. It costs a little more, but you will save money from making your own smoothies and from throwing the cheaper blenders away.

The Alchemy of Smoothies

The number of healthy ingredients available for smoothies is practically limitless, just by changing up the ingredients. Using different fruits and vegetables will help you get an even amount of nutrients and health benefits from the varying components. I try my best to use what's locally in season. If you're into green smoothies, be sure to rotate the greens every couple of weeks. This will also keep your smoothies new and exciting and prevent smoothie boredom. After your basic fruits and vegetables, you can add an array of the various spices, herbs, superfoods, and other health foods. The possibilities and combinations are endless.

Note* Avoid mixing melons with other produce, they don't mix well. You can make a melon smoothie but limit the produce to just melons.

Celery is great in smoothies, but if you don't have a Vitamix or other high end blender be sure to cut up the celery into tiny pieces to avoid the blades from damage.

To make a sweeter tasting smoothie, use a three to one formula. Three fruits to one vegetable.

For a vegetable based smoothie, use three vegetables and one fruit.

Start with a Healthy Base

There are many options you can use for your smoothies liquid base. You are only limited by your own imagination, have fun mixing fruits and vegetables, experiment!

Juice. If you are going to use juice, use only fresh-pressed, squeezed juice or 100% juice with no sugar added.

Water. If you are using only frozen fruits for your smoothie, use filtered drinking water as the liquid base to dilute the sweetness. Some people prefer a thinner consistency to their smoothie, so using a little bit of water can create the texture and consistency you need.

Coconut water. One of my favorite bases is water from a young (Thai) coconut, which provides sweetness and a bevy of electrolytes. Now a popular choice among athletes for post-workout recovery, coconut water can add a fresh flavor to your smoothies or shakes. Coconut water contains electrolytes and will rehydrate your body quickly and efficiently. You'll have more energy when you're not dehydrated.

Milk. I'm not a big fan of cow's milk but if you prefer to use milk, then try to go for skimmed milk instead.

Buttermilk. It's tangy but it can make a yummy compliment to some fruits and vegetables.

Fresh goat's milk. Goat's milk may cost more than cow's milk but is a healthier option.

Whole soy milk. This is another health drink that is made with polyunsaturated fats.

Avocado. Besides the nutrient content, avocados help add a creamy, smooth texture to smoothies. If you are not an avocado fan, add only one-half of an avocado to a smoothie — you'll barely taste it (yet still reap all the health benefits). Avocado. It's hard to beat the creamy texture of an avocado. Plus, it adds a dose of healthy fats, fiber, and potassium. In Brazil, avocado is commonly added to ice cream; why not make your smoothie a Brazilian ice cream treat?

Cottage cheese. Protein is important because it helps smoothies "stick with you" longer. Since protein takes longer to digest, it keeps you from getting hungry too soon. Sure, you can reach for the protein powder, but that's often expensive and can give your drink a gritty taste. Cottage cheese contains 15 grams of protein in half a cup, and it adds a creamy texture that you can't get from plain yogurt, milk, or soy milk.

Ricotta cheese. It is almost always made from cow's milk in the USA, but in Italy it is also made from sheep, goat and even water buffalo milk. Ricotta boasts healthful benefits through its protein, fat and vitamin and mineral contents.

Yogurt. Most people who are lactose intolerant are able to stomach yogurt, the healthier option to be included into your smoothie. Choose Greek plain (unflavored) yogurt for optimum health benefit. If you buy yogurt in small containers, you can freeze these and use these in your smoothies too.

Frozen yogurts, choose wisely, but always go for low-fat or non-fat where possible. Vanilla or plain flavor is a common favorite.

Non-dairy milks. Going with a dairy alternative for the liquid portion of your smoothie is a great way to mix things up, and can provide you with different tastes and nutrient combos. Hemp Bliss milk comes in a few different flavors, both sweetened and unsweetened, and has calcium and omega-3 fats. And if you have allergy issues, rice milk is a great option.

Nut or seed milk. You can purchase these from your local health food stores or you can make your own nut milk at home.

Homemade Nut Milk

Place 1 c. raw, unsalted (preferably organic!) almonds in a bowl and cover with water. Cover and soak overnight on counter. Drain and rinse really well. Place in high speed blender along with 3-4 cups filtered water (depending on your preference of consistency). Blend approx. 45 seconds. Strain into a pitcher using a nut milk bag (this takes a little time to get all the liquid but is well worth the effort). Once pulp is completely wrung dry, replace almond milk back into blender and add 2 1/2 tsp. vanilla, 1/2 tsp. cinnamon and whatever natural sweetener you like honey, agave, and stevia, to add to the taste. I use a 1/2 c. of a homemade concoction of coconut water from one "young" coconut and about 8 pitted dates, soaked in coconut water overnight in the refrigerator. Next day I pop them in the blender. Freeze for longer or store in refrigerator for up to 5 days. This makes your almond milk not only extremely delicious, but it's adding electrolytes as well.

Cashew Almond Milk

1 cup boiling water

1 cup raw cashews

1 cup ice

1 vanilla bean, seeds scraped (reserve the bean itself for another use), or 1 teaspoon pure vanilla extract

1 tablespoon agave nectar

This will stay in the refrigerator up to one week, or freeze up to 6 months.

Coffee. Need a pick me up? Coffee can be added to your smoothie. You can add instant granules or brew your coffee and let it cool before you add it to your smoothie.

Tea. Using a healthy or medicinal tea can really improve the nutrition of your smoothie. In some circles "elixir" is the term used to designate these drinks. Use a healthy tea instead of water, milk, or juice as the base of your smoothie to boost the nutrition. This is wonderful for its anti-oxidant properties. Steep the leaves/sachets in boiled water for about 4 to 5 minutes, strain the leaves and leave it to cool before using for your smoothie. I often make a large pot of medicinal tea on the weekend and store in half gallon mason jars for use during the week.

If you're working on a particular health issue there's almost certainly an herb, if not several, that can help address that issue and would be a great tea candidate. Even something as simple as green tea is great place to start.

Kombucha tea near other refrigerated teas in natural foods stores and well-stocked supermarkets. Kombucha is available in many different flavors.

Kefir. It's a fermented milk drink made with milk from cows, goats or sheep, and many people find it easier to digest than whole milk. You can also look for kefir made from soy or other dairy alternatives. Kefir is a drinkable yogurt found in the dairy section of most supermarkets, it supplies a healthy amount of protein and calcium and good-for-you probiotics.

Tofu. Is a good source of protein. It is tasteless, but it does add a rich and creamy texture to your smoothie. I prefer to use the silken type, it's creamy.

White beans. An unusual smoothie ingredient, to be sure, but beans are arguably one of the most nutritious foods out there. Many Americans rarely eat them, which is a shame, since beans are the only food that count as both a vegetable and a meat substitute because of their diverse nutrients. They'll add fiber, protein, iron, and potassium to your smoothie. White beans are easiest to "hide" in a light-colored smoothie, while darker beans work best in dark drinks.

Smoothie Flavorings

There are many natural flavorings you can add to your smoothie to give it that extra kick, especially when your main ingredients are mainly vegetable base, you may want to sweeten it up a little to make it more palatable.

Use natural sweeteners like raisins, fruit juice concentrate (be careful of added sugar), raw honey, maple syrup, stevia, molasses and dates. Using dates or raisins is a great way to sweeten your smoothie. Be sure to remove the pits and soak them overnight or for at least an hour before blending. I recommend other options such as stevia products, stevia comes in many different flavors like English toffee, or vanilla. You can also use xylitol in small amounts or glucose which is sold as dextrose and can easily be purchased in most health food stores.

Various coconut products (shreds, flakes, raw meat, oil, butter)

Jelly can add a wonderful naturally sweet flavor to your smoothie. It is best to use a natural seedless variety in any flavor you love.

Fresh ginger or ginger juice (use only 1 teaspoon at any time) gives your smoothie the added spice and powerful anti-oxidants. With ginger's ability to kill ovarian cancer cells and relieve nausea and inflammation, why not include it? Just a 1/2 teaspoon of freshly grated ginger to your smoothie concoction can go a long way. To make ginger juice, boil one cup of water and add one small piece of ginger to the water, let it steep for 5 minutes or longer, depending on how strong of a ginger flavor you desire.

Spice it up. Various spices enhance both flavor and nutrition. Play with them and perfect the taste. You can also adjust the taste, and healthiness, of your smoothie by using common spices. Cinnamon, vanilla, ginger, nutmeg, and cayenne are a few of my favorites. One challenge of the perfect smoothie is achieving the right sweetness, without overloading on sugar. Enter cinnamon—it adds a layer of sweetness, with no calories at all. Plus, studies show that cinnamon may be helpful at managing your cholesterol and blood sugar levels. German researchers found that cinnamon can lower blood sugar by 10 percent in type 2 diabetics. Cinnamon compounds trigger insulin receptors for more favorable blood-sugar levels.

Cardamom. An ancient digestion aid that can ease stomach cramps and flatulence, cardamom also triggers the release of bile that will help your body break down fat faster. You can add ground cardamom to your smoothies or look for organic chai tea bags that include cardamom spice. You can sweeten with honey and a splash of organic milk for a tasty smoothie.

Cloves: A go-to home remedy for toothaches, cloves also contain eugenol, a compound that activates insulin production to help regulate blood-sugar levels. The spice is also a potent source of manganese, a trace mineral that helps build tissue and bones. People with low manganese levels are more prone to arthritis.

To use it in your smoothie, steep in your cup of tea and then add it to your smoothie.

Coriander: Aromatic and medicinal, this spice has been shown to ease anxiety and help people sleep. It's also an important spice for people living with type 2 diabetes. This spice works best when using avocados, tomatoes and greens.

Need something salty? Adding a high quality salt to your smoothie not only provides much needed minerals, but also perfects the taste. A dash of a high quality salt will increase the minerals and improve the taste of your smoothie. I prefer Celtic sea salt. There are a plethora of good salts to choose from, just make sure to avoid nutritionally bankrupt white table salt. Try dried Kelp Flakes, for a little taste of salt from the ocean.

Super Food Add-Ins

The list below is not meant to overwhelm you, but rather give you an idea of what's possible, and available. This is not a complete list of superfoods to add to your smoothie, but it's a good place to start. You're on your way to becoming a smoothie alchemist so experiment and try different superfoods to really boost the nutrition of your smoothie.

Here's a list of examples of other powdered supplements which you may add to your healthful smoothies (these are blended together with your other ingredients). Read the label for dosage. Check with your physician before adding any supplements to your diet, some supplements may react with medications.

Acai. Acai contains several substances called anthocyanins and flavonoids. Anthocyanins and flavonoids are powerful antioxidants that help defend the body against life's stressors. They also play a role in the body's cell protection system. Free radicals are harmful byproducts produced by the body. Eating a diet rich in antioxidants may interfere with aging and the disease process by neutralizing free radicals. By lessening the destructive power of free radicals, antioxidants may help reduce the risk of some diseases, such as heart disease and cancer.

Astragalus Root may help protect the body from diseases such as cancer and diabetes. It contains antioxidants, which protect cells against damage caused by free radicals, byproducts of cellular energy. Astragalus is used to protect and support the immune system, for preventing colds and upper respiratory infections, to lower blood pressure, to treat diabetes, and to protect the liver. It helps ward off bacterial and viral infections to boost immunity -- a must if you're tired or stressed. Use 200 to 400 mg (or 1 to 2 teaspoons of alcohol-free extract) but be sure to read the label for exact dosage.

Banana powder. If you want the potassium of bananas without the bulk of adding them whole, try using banana powder instead. It's made from dried bananas finely milled, and its potassium can act like a natural energy drink after a tough workout.

Barley grass. Barley grass has 11 times more calcium than cow's milk, 5 times more iron than spinach and 7 times more Vitamin C and bio-flavonoids than orange juice. It contains significant amounts of Vitamin B12 which is very important in a vegetarian diet. Barley grass juice has anti-viral activities and neutralizes heavy metals such as mercury in the blood.

Bee pollen. Bee pollen contains vitamins, minerals, carbohydrates, lipids, and protein. It comes from the pollen that collects on the bodies of bees. Bee pollen may also include bee saliva. It's important to avoid confusing bee pollen with natural honey, honeycomb, bee venom, or royal jelly. These products do not contain bee pollen.

Brewer's yeast. Brewer's yeast is used for diarrhea, the common cold and other upper respiratory tract infections, influenza, swine flu, acne, premenstrual syndrome, and type 2 diabetes. It has also been used as a source of B vitamins, chromium, and protein.

Cacao. Research shows that cacao is full of antioxidants called flavonoids, which can also improve heart health. Keep in mind that cacao nibs are bitterer than cacao powder.

Calcium powder. This is a hypoallergenic formulation of calcium powder with vitamin D that has been specially designed for individuals with special requirements and sensitivities.

Chlorella powder. Chlorella is a good source of protein, fats, carbohydrates, fiber, chlorophyll, vitamins, and minerals. Chlorella is a fresh water algae and like its other algae cousins contains a complete protein profile, all the B vitamins, vitamin C and E and many minerals. It is amazing for the immune system and for reducing cholesterol and preventing the hardening of the arteries, a precursor to heart attacks and strokes.

Chia. Chia is a gluten-free ancient grain that can be added to just about any food. Chia stabilizes blood sugars, manages the effects of diabetes, improves insulin sensitivity and aids symptoms related to metabolic syndrome, including imbalances in cholesterol, blood pressure and high blood sugar after meals. Try soaking your chia seeds in a little water to make a gel that gives your smoothie a nice smooth consistency.

Coconut oil. Studies have shown that intake of coconut oil can help our bodies mount resistance to both viruses and bacteria that can cause illness. Even more, it also can help to fight off yeast, fungus and candida. Coconut oil can also positively affect our hormones for thyroid and blood sugar control. People who take coconut oil also tend to have improvements in how they handle blood sugar since coconut can help improve insulin use within the body. Coconut oil can boost thyroid function helping to increase metabolism, energy and endurance. It increases digestion and helps to absorb fat-soluble vitamins. A good fat like coconut, flax, or hemp oil, an avocado, or cream will keep you satiated and full of energy for hours, and put the smooth in smoothie.

Cooked brown rice or unpolished rice. You can purchase brown or unpolished rice (more fibrous and less starchy) from your local health food store. Cook it and leave to cool before use.

Echinacea. Echinacea is a household name when it comes to warding off colds and flu. This herb is used as a natural antibiotic and immune system stimulator, helping to build up resistance. The reason for its effectiveness is because of its ability to stimulate the lymph flow in the body. Lymph runs parallel with our bloodstream and carries toxins out of the body. The herb can be purchased in a liquid form to add to your smoothie.

Fish Oils. Omega's fatty acids, these fatty acids have been linked to helping prevent heart disease, cancer, and many other diseases. Taking omega-3 fish oils could help to protect against skin cancer. Some fish oil capsules can taste and smell fishy, this could ruin the taste of your smoothie, so be sure to read the labels to identify which brands don't smell fishy. Open up the capsule and squeeze oil into your smoothie.

Flax. Flax is full of lignans phytoestrogenic compounds that have been proven to help protect us against certain kinds of cancers, especially breast, prostate and colon. Adding two to three tablespoons of flaxseeds to your smoothies daily can reduce your cancer risk and also provide a dose of four grams of fiber and essential fatty acids. The oils in flaxseeds can go rancid quickly, so be sure to purchase ground flaxseed in a vacuum-sealed package and store them in the freezer. Better yet, you can grind your own daily. Studies have shown that the omega-3 fats and high concentrations of fiber found in flaxseed may reduce inflammation in the joints and help fight against diabetes and heart disease. Flaxseeds also contain natural, cancer-protective compounds known as liganans, which can prevent the development of colon and breast cancer and strengthen the body's ability to defend itself against bacteria and viruses. Add ground flaxseeds to your smoothie rather than whole ones to ensure successful absorption.

Goji berries. Berries like the goji berry are filled with powerful antioxidants and other compounds that may help prevent cancer and other illnesses, including heart disease. Antioxidants may also boost the immune system and lower cholesterol.

Ginseng. Ginseng is the quintessential herb for handling stress. This ancient healing herb has been used widely throughout Asia as an energizer tonic. This special herb is particularly beneficial when recovering from illness or surgery for its restorative and anti-infection properties. It promotes regeneration from stress and fatigue. Several human studies have also shown that ginseng may lower blood sugar levels, which could benefit people with type 2 diabetes. Of course, people with diabetes should only take ginseng under the care of a doctor.

Green Superfood powders increase nutrition of your smoothie in a hurry. You can find this at your local health food store.

Hemp seeds/protein. Hemp is considered one of the world's most nutritious plants. Hemp seeds contain all of the essential amino acids making them an ideal source of protein for vegans and raw foodists. The essential fatty acids are abundant in hemp seeds and come in a ratio that is highly beneficial to humans. Magnesium, iron, and potassium are in good supply along with fiber. Some of hemp seed's supply of antioxidants comes from its vitamin E content.

Kelp. Kelp is considered a super-food because of all the nutrients it contains. Kelp contains many vitamins, especially B vitamins, which are essential for cellular metabolism and providing your body with energy. It also contains vitamins C and E, which are both strong antioxidants and promote blood vessel health. Minerals, such as calcium, boron and magnesium are plentiful in kelp; they are necessary for strong bones and normal muscle function.

Lecithin powder or granules. Lecithin can increase your body's acetylcholine levels, helping to guard against memory loss. Try adding 1 to 2 grams (1 to 2 level tablespoons) of granular or liquid lecithin.

Liquid vitamins. If your kids hate to take their vitamins, this is an easy way for them to get their vitamins. Be sure to read the bottle for the recommended dosage per child.

Maca. is a Peruvian root plant that is slightly sweet and has been shown to increase energy, endurance, and improve sexual function. The best form for smoothies is when it's in a raw, powdered state. When using maca for the first time, start with a tablespoon of powder since the flavor is quite distinctive. If you'd like to add more, a banana or berries can instantly mask the taste.

Mushroom Power. Boost your immune system with mushroom powders like Reishi, Cordyceps, and Maitake. Just open a capsule or two and dump in your smoothie.

Nettle - the bowel mover. These plants are best known as stinging nettle plants. However when the nettle leaves are dried and eaten the saliva neutralizes the sting. Nettles are incredibly effective in removing unwanted pounds. The best way to add nettle to your smoothie is to make a cup of nettle tea, let it cool before you add it to your other ingredients. Check with your doctor before offering this to children.

Noni. This fruit has been used by Polynesian islanders as a regenerative medicine for more than 1500 years. Research documents that the noni fruit has astounding anti-bacterial properties, even against E-coli. It has anti-tumor activity, anti-inflammatory properties, is effective as a pain reliever, generates cell repair and strengthens the immune system. Noni contains a multitude of vitamins, minerals, enzymes and phytonutrients. Many believe that the synergistic effect of the multi-spectrum nutrients is what gives it its potency. It has been proven beneficial for colds and flu's, digestive disorders, skin disorders, pain relief, headaches, infections and more. For best results look for a freeze-dried product that uses only the whole fruit or when buying the juice look for a brand that does not use pasteurizing.

Nuts. Any kind of nuts: Finely grind any kind of nuts (almonds, cashew nuts, hazelnuts, peanuts, pecans, etc.) to be added to your smoothies for the thick smooth taste and health properties only nuts provide. You can add smoothies in your drink or on top of your smoothie.

Oats. Oats have a higher level of soluble fiber and are helpful in lowering cholesterol level. Eaten on its own, oats may taste rather bland, so add it to your smoothie. Let it stand in hot boiled water and leave to cool before use.

Peanut butter. With its high levels of monounsaturated fats, peanut butter provides protection against heart diseases. When buying peanut butter, check that the ingredients do not contain hydrogenated vegetable oils which are rich in trans-fatty acids. Add peanut butter to the kids' smoothies' recipes, they will love it!

Powdered milk. There are a variety of non-fat powdered milk forms.

Sesame Seed. The nutrients in sesame seeds are better absorbed when ground. Add some sesame seeds into your smoothie for its anti-oxidant properties.

Spirulina is a cultivated micro-algae which has been consumed for thousands of years by the indigenous peoples in Mexico and Africa. It is one of the highest known protein sources on Earth and contains 70% complete protein, towering over steak which consists of only 25% protein once cooked. Studies have shown that spirulina can help control blood sugar levels and cravings thus making it a key food for diabetics, and can be used to assist in weight loss and as a general nutritional supplement. Spirulina and chlorella powder are amazing sources of almost every vitamin and are 70% protein by weight; they will also turn your smoothie green!

Vitamin C powder. Vitamin C is a natural antioxidant and immune booster. Try adding 200 mg of powdered vitamin C or crushed chewable vitamin C tablets.

Vitamin E can nourish the skin, help maintain healthy cholesterol levels, and ease symptoms of peri-menopause. Add 400 IU of vitamin E or 80 mg of tocopherols and tocotrienols. Squeeze gelcaps to release liquid into the smoothie.

Wheat bran. Wheat bran is beneficial toward providing digestive regularity and ending constipation because it is very high in dietary fiber. Some also claim that foods containing bran provide a feeling of fullness. This claim may be true, since it tends to absorb water and expand in the digestive system.

Wheat Germ. Wheat germ is packed with good nutrients. Two tablespoons of raw wheat germ have about 1.5 grams of unsaturated fat, 9 grams of carbohydrates, and 4 grams of protein, 2 grams dietary fiber, 2 grams of sugars, no cholesterol and about 60 calories.

Wheat Grass Powder. Wheat grass is the sprouted grass of a wheat seed. Unlike the whole grain, because it has been sprouted, it no longer contains gluten or other common allergic agents. Wheat grass is super alkalizing and is excellent for promoting healthy blood. It normalizes the thyroid gland to stimulate metabolism thus assisting digestion and promoting weight loss due also to its high enzyme content and cleansing effect. Unless you have a Vitamix or Blendtec, wheat grass doesn't get blended as well and will leaves little pieces of grass behind. Therefore, to get the benefits of wheat grass you can now buy it in powder form at local health food stores.

Whey Protein. As a pure, natural and high quality protein from cow's milk, whey protein is a rich source of essential amino acids, the building blocks for healthy muscles, skin and other body tissue. Its high levels of leucine preserve lean muscle tissue and promote fat loss, making this powdery substance a perfect addition to a smoothie. You can add protein powder or you can add other types of food that contain more protein such as nuts, seeds, quinoa, grains such as oats, sprouted seeds or beans, tofu, or other dairy free forms of protein. Bear in mind that greens contain a high level of protein per gram, you just need to eat more of it to get the same amount of protein. I also add oats to get enough carbs to keep my kids fueled up and filled up until the next meal. You would be feeling full with the added fiber, complex carbohydrates, healthy monounsaturated fats and fat-soluble vitamins.

Wild blue-green algae. Algae was the first form of life on Earth and its power is immense. Wild blue-green algae is a phyto-plankton and contains virtually every nutrient. With a 60% protein content and a more complete amino acid profile than beef or soy beans. It contains one of the best known food sources of beta carotene, B vitamins and chlorophyll. It has been shown to improve brain function and memory, strengthen the immune system and help with viruses, colds and flu.

Smoothie Science

Learning how to make a smoothie is actually pretty easy if you follow the steps below.

Step 1: Pick a Smoothie Recipe

Choose a smoothie recipe you would like to make based on your personal goals; good health, weight loss, more energy, mental clarity, relaxation, muscle builder, or a smoothie that just sounds delicious. Many nutritionists recommend that you have at least 4-5 green smoothies per week. My kids and I have had a smoothie every day for the past 15 years in addition I use Mondays as my big smoothie day. I will have a red or yellow smoothie for breakfast and a green smoothie for lunch, for dinner I will have a bowl of vegetable soup, I call this my maintenance program, I am proud to say I am the same weight now as I was in college.

Step 2: Add Your Liquid

The first thing to add into your blender is the liquid, which is usually around 1 to 2 cups. Follow what your smoothie recipe calls for, but keep a few things in mind. The more liquid you add, the more watery or runnier your smoothie will be. Some people like it this way. If you prefer a thicker consistency, use slightly less liquid.

Step 3: Add Your Base

The "base" is what will provide a creamy smoothie texture. Think of it as the "body" of your smoothie. Many smoothie recipes call for a banana or two. Bananas are a terrific base and provide your smoothie with a nice creaminess, and sweet taste. Fruits such as mango, peach, pear and apple will also do the trick. Other good options include avocado, coconut meat, chia seed gel, nut butters, yogurt, frozen fruit and ice.

Water rich fruits like watermelon and pineapple won't give you that creamy smoothie consistency. If you are looking for a way to save calories bulk u on denser smoothies and eliminate ice. Adding ice is a quick and easy way to thicken a smoothie full of water laden fruits.

Step 4: Add Fruits and/or Vegetables

Now that you've got your liquid and base squared away, it's time to add the fruits and/or vegetables the smoothie recipe you're making calls for.

This is also a great time to experiment, get creative, and have fun exploring the various fruit and vegetable combinations your taste buds adore. Most fruit can be used either fresh or frozen, see which you prefer. If you're making a green smoothie with the likes of spinach, kale, beet greens, dandelion greens, arugula, or lettuce, you may want to cut the greens into smaller pieces depending on the power of your blender. You also may want to add the greens into your blender last, after adding any optional add-ins.

Step 5: Superfood Add-ins

This is where you can use your smoothie alchemist skills and take your smoothie to the next level of nutrition and tastiness, and have lots of fun doing so. As your smoothie skills develop, you'll intuitively know which add-ins to use in which recipes.

Some of the best superfood add-ins are:

2 T flaxseeds

2 T chia seeds

Chopped nuts

1/4 cup coconut flakes or shreds

1 serving of your preferred protein and/or green superfood powder

ICE WHEN? Always add the ice last. Otherwise you may over blend the ice and it will make your smoothie watery rather than frosty and icy like we all love. Crushed ice is best. The easiest way to crush ice is in a plastic bag with a rolling pin.

Step 6: Blend It Up!

Now that you've added all your lovely ingredients into your blender, it's show time. Depending on your blender, and smoothie ingredients, you may need to start out on a low setting (or pulse) before getting up to top blending speed. Some blenders even come with a handy smoothie button for extra easy smoothie making. I like to blend my smoothies until the liquid is fully circulating within the blender for about 5 seconds. Total blend time is usually between 30 to 60 seconds depending on the ingredients. It may take you a few blends to get it down, puree until smooth and thoroughly mixed, scraping down sides with rubber spatula as necessary.

Divide among glasses. Serve immediately or store in the refrigerator. If refrigerating, whisk to recombine just before serving.

Smoothie Troubleshooting

Here are a few of the common smoothie making mishaps people often experience along with the remedy.

Is your smoothie too frothy? Try using a little less liquid, and make sure not to blend too long. Try withholding the liquid (maybe just half) until the other ingredients are thoroughly mixed or liquefied, then add the remaining liquid and only blend on the lowest speed until it's incorporated.

The thickening or "base" ingredients mentioned above (banana, avocado, coconut meat, chia seed gel, nut butter, yogurt, frozen fruit and ice) will help. Milk can cause frothiness, maybe try organic apple juice or water instead. When blending greens like baby spinach, you won't need as much liquid because they blend so well and contain a fair amount themselves.

Is your smoothie to runny? The quick fix for this is reducing the amount of liquid. More thickening smoothie ingredients will also alleviate this problem.

Is your smoothie not tasty or sweet enough? Simply add a little more of your preferred sweetener. I recommend honey, stevia, maple syrup, and dates.

Is your green smoothie too bitter? Use less greens and/or more sweet fruit and sweetener.

Is your smoothie not blending very well? Filling your blender jar to high might result in less than ideal blending. If you have an older or low powered blender, you may need to blend your liquid, base, fresh fruit, and greens (chop into small pieces) first, then add in any frozen fruit or ice cubes and blend until nice and smooth. You may also need to add more liquid to balance out the ingredients. Your blender may be the culprit. You may have an older, less powerful, blender that simply can't get the job done.

Consuming your smoothies:

Eat/drink your smoothies within 10 minutes of making them to take full advantage of the nutrients before they oxidize and turn your smoothie brown. I do not recommend storing smoothies after it has gone through the blender as once the fruits/vegetables are cut up in the blender, the nutrients and live enzymes will deteriorate rapidly.

The Formula's

Below is a list of ingredients to make delicious healthy smoothies. The directions are the same so please refer to The 6 steps, (page 39) to make a smoothie. I have not added the ½ cup of ice to every recipe, I personally don't add it, but you may, so if you are going to add ice, be sure its crushed ice.

Most of the following recipes are approximately 2-3 servings. Remember to add your Super food Add-ins.

Red/Orange Smoothies

Dreams

1 cup vanilla frozen yogurt

1 cup orange juice

1 orange peel and pith removed, cut into chunks

Blend until smooth

Small Joys

1 cup Greek yogurt

1 cup raspberries

½ cup non-fat milk, almond milk, soy milk

½ cup ice cubes

Blend until smooth

Super Angel

1 cup vanilla-flavored soy milk

Smoothies! Become a Smoothie Alchemist

¼ cup orange juice

1 T local honey

½ cup mango

½ cup frozen strawberries

Blend until smooth

Youthful Wisdom

1 cup coconut milk

½ cup soft silken tofu

2 T local honey

2 T chia seed

1 cup frozen blueberries

Blend until smooth

Intelligent Choice

1 cup carrot juice

1 orange, skin removed

2 T flaxseed

2 T local honey

1 tsp. ground allspice

½ cup crushed ice

Blend until smooth

Smoothies! Become a Smoothie Alchemist

Peak Performance

1 banana

1 8 ounce can crushed pineapple use the juice too

1cup vanilla yogurt

1 cup orange juice

Blend until smooth

Beautiful Eyes

3 medium carrots, peeled and sliced (1-1/2 cups)

1 ½ cups apple juice

½ avocado

Blend until smooth

Wisdom

1 grapefruit, peeled, seeded, and chopped

2 cups frozen strawberries

1 sweet apple cored and chopped

1 inch fresh ginger, peeled and chopped

1 cup cold filtered water

Blend until smooth

Naturally Beautiful

1 cup yogurt

Smoothies! Become a Smoothie Alchemist

1 banana

2 cups strawberries

1 cup orange juice

Blend until smooth

New Light

1 peach

1 mango

1 banana

1 cup Greek yogurt

1 cup orange juice

Blend until smooth

Natural Vitamins

1 banana

1/2 cup bottled carrot juice

1/2 cup plain yogurt

3/4-inch piece peeled fresh ginger, coarsely chopped

½ cup crushed ice

Blend until smooth

Healthy for Life

2 1/2 cups papaya chunks

Smoothies! Become a Smoothie Alchemist

2/3 cup plain Greek yogurt

1 T finely chopped peeled fresh ginger

1 T local honey

Juice of 2 lemons

16 fresh mint leaves

½ cup crushed ice

Blend until smooth

Wellness Formula

1 mango (or 1 1/2 cups frozen mango chunks)

1 cup carrot juice

1 tsp. nutmeg

1/2 cup ice cubes (omit if using frozen mango)

Blend until smooth

Respect Yourself

1 cup frozen pitted cherries

3/4 cup pomegranate juice

1 cup plain Greek yogurt

1 T local honey

1 tsp. lemon juice

1 tsp. of cinnamon

1 tsp. of salt

Smoothies! Become a Smoothie Alchemist

2 cups crushed ice

Blend until smooth

Powerful Immune System

4 tangerines, peeled

2 limes, juice and zest

¼ cup local honey

1 cup crushed ice

Blend until smooth

Open Your Heart

1 cup frozen strawberries

1 cup soymilk

1 banana

1/4 cup local honey

1 package silken soft tofu

2 T fresh lemon juice

Pinch of salt

Blend until smooth

Soulful

1 cup frozen raspberries

1 cup almond milk

Smoothies! Become a Smoothie Alchemist

1 cup frozen pitted cherries

2 T local honey

1 tsp. flaxseed

½ lemon squeeze juice

Blend until smooth

Power of the Heart

¾ cup papaya

¾ cup peaches

1 pear

1 tsp. fresh ginger peeled and chopped

2 mint leaves

½ cup filtered water

½ cup crushed ice

Blend until smooth

Healthy on the Inside

1 cup strawberries

1 cup strawberry non-fat yogurt

1/8 cup finely chopped blanched almonds

1 cup un-sweetened apple juice

1 cup apricot nectar

Blend until smooth

Smoothies! Become a Smoothie Alchemist

Mind-Body

1 cup raspberries

1 orange

1 cup orange juice

1 cup Greek plain yogurt

Blend until smooth

Fulfillment

1/2 cup of mango

1/2 cup of papaya

Juice of 1 orange

1/2 cup of carrot juice

1 small piece of fresh ginger, peeled and chopped

½ cup crushed ice

Blend until smooth

Courage

2 cups strawberries

1 1/2 cups milk

¼ cup maple syrup

¼ cup wheat germ

1 tsp. ground cinnamon

1 1/2 cups crushed ice

Smoothies! Become a Smoothie Alchemist

Blend until smooth

Love

1 1/4 cups vegetable juice, chilled

1/2 peeled cucumber

3 kale leaves

1 lemon-squeeze the juice

Blend until smooth

Conscious Eating

1 cup acai berry juice

1 cup mango

1 orange peeled and segmented

2 cups crushed ice

Blend until smooth

Goodness Gracious

4 cups cubed seeded watermelon

1 lime juice plus zest

1T xylitol or other sweetener

1 cup filtered water

Blend until smooth

Smoothies! Become a Smoothie Alchemist

Alive!

1 peach

1 cup strawberries

1 cup Greek yogurt

½ cup peach nectar

Blend until smooth

Concentration

1 cup strawberries

1 cup pineapple chunks

1/2 cup raspberries

2 T frozen limeade

1 cup Greek plain yogurt

1 cup orange juice

Blend until smooth

Zen

1/3 cup of blueberries

1/3 cup of raspberries

1/3 cup of pomegranate arials

1/4 cup of beet juice

1 banana

1 cup Pomegranate juice

Smoothies! Become a Smoothie Alchemist

1 1/2 cups fresh raspberries

6 T frozen limeade concentrate

1 cup crushed ice

2 sprigs fresh mint

Blend until smooth

Love My Family

1/2 cup frozen raspberries

1/2 cup plain Greek yogurt

1 banana

1/2 cup old-fashioned rolled oats

1 T local honey

1 cup coconut water

½ cup crushed ice

Blend until smooth

Sweetness of Life

1 cup strawberries

1 cup vanilla flavored Greek yogurt

5 basil leaves

1 T lime juice

1 tsp. agave syrup

Blend until smooth

Smoothies! Become a Smoothie Alchemist

Forever Young

1 ¼ cup apple juice

2 cups cantaloupe

½ cup crushed ice

Blend until smooth

Honor Health

1 ½ cups strawberries

1 cup frozen unsweetened pitted dark sweet cherries

1 cup fresh raspberries

1 cup pomegranate juice, chilled

½ cup fresh blueberries

Blend until smooth

Incredible Me

2 cups chopped cantaloupe

1 lime juice and zest

1 T local honey

1 cup filtered water

½ cup crushed ice

Blend until smooth

Smoothies! Become a Smoothie Alchemist

Pomegranate Surprise

1 cup pomegranate juice

Arials from a pomegranate (surprise)

1 cup vanilla Greek yogurt

2 tablespoons honey

Blend until smooth

Interconnectedness

1 1/4 cups tomato juice

1/4 cup carrot juice

1/2 peeled cucumber

1/2 celery stalk (be sure to chop into small pieces)

¼ cup parsley

¼ cup spinach

1/2 cup crushed ice

Blend until smooth

Essential Nutrition

1 cup frozen yogurt

1 cup raspberries

2 nectarines, stone removed

½ cup almond milk

1 tsp. local honey

Smoothies! Become a Smoothie Alchemist

Blend until smooth

Heart of Nutrition

1 cup raspberries

¾ cup chilled almond or rice milk

¼ cup frozen pitted unsweetened cherries

1 ½ T honey

2 tsp. finely grated fresh ginger

1 tsp. ground flaxseed

Squeeze of fresh lemon juice

Blend until smooth

Heavenly Being

1 cup frozen strawberries

1 cup of frozen raspberries

1 cup of frozen mango

1 ½ cups of orange juice

Blend until smooth

Reflection

1 cup blood orange juice

1 cup vanilla yogurt

1 banana

A little honey, maple syrup, or stevia to sweeten (optional)

Blend until smooth

Strong & Fit

1/2 cup each pumpkin puree

½ cup silken tofu

3 1/2 tablespoons maple syrup

1 cup milk (any type)

1/2 teaspoon pumpkin pie spice

½ tsp. sea salt

½ cup crushed ice

Blend until smooth

Karma

1/2 cup pineapple chunks juice too (you can use a can)

1 banana

1/2 cup frozen raspberries

1 T local honey

1/4 cup carrot juice

1/2 cup vanilla soy milk

1/2 cup freshly squeezed orange juice

Blend until smooth

Garden of Healthy Eating

2 cups freshly squeezed orange juice (about 6 oranges)

1/4 cup local honey

1 T freshly squeezed lemon juice

2 tsp. finely grated fresh ginger

2 frozen bananas

Blend until smooth

Laughter

1 cup strawberries

½ cup rolled oats

1 cup Greek yogurt

1 cup almond milk

2 T flax seed

½ cup crushed ice

Blend until smooth

Buzz

2 cups frozen peach slices

1 cup carrot juice

1 cup orange juice

2 T ground flaxseed

1 T chopped fresh ginger

Smoothies! Become a Smoothie Alchemist

Blend until smooth

Blueprint of Life

1 cup frozen vanilla yogurt

1 1/2 cups frozen pitted cherries

1/2 tsp. vanilla extract,

1/4 tsp. almond extract

Blend until smooth

Lighten Up

4 peaches (about 1 pound) or canned

½ cup silken tofu

1/3 cup freshly squeezed orange juice

1 T local honey

Blend until smooth

Mother Nature

1 cup carrot juice

1 green apple

2 tsp. freshly grated ginger

1 cup freshly squeezed orange juice

1 tablespoon honey

Blend until smooth

Yellow/Beige Smoothies

Friendship

1 banana

1/2 cup Greek yogurt

1/2 cup milk

1/4 cup old-fashioned rolled oats

2 tsp. flaxseeds

1 T local honey

½ cups crushed ice

Blend until smooth

Pure & Clean

4 Swiss chard leaves

1 banana

1 peach

¼ cup pineapple

¼ cup hazelnuts

½ avocado

½ cup crushed ice

Blend until smooth

Smoothies! Become a Smoothie Alchemist

You are Pear-fect

1 1/2 cups Greek yogurt

1 pear, chopped

1 banana

2 T protein powder

½ cup crushed ice

Blend until smooth

Hawaiian Health

1- 8 ounce can pineapple chunks, juice too

1 mango

1 banana

1 cup pineapple yogurt

½ cup crushed ice

Blend until smooth

Air

1 nectarine, remove skin

1 cup milk (any type)

1 cup pineapple yogurt

½ cup crushed ice

Blend until smooth

Smoothies! Become a Smoothie Alchemist

Serendipity

2 cups frozen sliced peaches

1 1/2 cups buttermilk

3 T maple syrup

1 T grated fresh ginger

½ cup crushed ice

Blend until smooth

Health from the Sun

1 cup pineapple yogurt

1 cup fat-free milk

1 banana

1 cup mango

½ cup crushed ice

Blend until smooth

Cheerful

1 cup pineapple

1 cup mango

1 cup coconut water

1 tsp. ground allspice

½ cup crushed ice

Blend until smooth

Smoothies! Become a Smoothie Alchemist

Sprinkle with toasted coconut

Glowing

2 tsp. Poppy seeds

1 lemon juice and zest

1 cup plain Greek yogurt

1/2 cup almond milk

1 cup crushed ice

Blend until smooth

Pure Happiness

2 cups frozen coconut water

2 cups each chopped pineapple

1 1/2 tablespoons lime juice

1 T local honey

1/2 cup coconut water

Blend until smooth

Love Myself

2 grapefruits segmented

2 T stevia or xylitol

1 tsp. cinnamon

1 cup crushed ice

Smoothies! Become a Smoothie Alchemist

Blend until smooth

Natural High

1 1/2 cups apricot nectar

1/2 cup vanilla Greek yogurt

2 T almond butter

½ cup crushed ice

Blend until smooth

Thanks-for-Giving

1 banana

1/3 cup cold canned pumpkin (not pie mix)

1/3 cup fat-free (skim) milk

1/4 cup plain Greek Yogurt

1 T frozen orange juice concentrate

2 tsp. Maple Syrup

½ tsp. ground cinnamon

½ tsp. ground nutmeg

Blend until smooth

Nurture Yourself

1 banana

¼ cup rolled oats

Smoothies! Become a Smoothie Alchemist

1 cup Greek yogurt

1 tsp. local honey

½ cup skim milk

1 tsp. of cinnamon

Blend until smooth

Circle of Life

¼ cup white beans

1 cup vanilla low-fat Greek yogurt

1 cup vanilla almond milk

1 tsp. vanilla extract or stevia

2 tsp. maple syrup

Blend until smooth

Peace

1 apple

1/2-inch fresh minced ginger

2 limes juice plus zest

1/4 cup honey

1 cup filtered water

2 cups crushed ice

Blend until smooth

Smoothies! Become a Smoothie Alchemist

Powerful Health

2 bananas

2 cups vanilla kefir

1/2 tsp. Ground cinnamon

1/8 tsp. Ground nutmeg

1/8 tsp. Ground allspice

Blend until smooth

Sunshine

2 cups diced frozen mango

1 1/2 cups pineapple juice

3/4 cup silken tofu

1/4 cup lime juice

1 tsp. freshly grated lime zest

Blend until smooth

Almond Delight

1 ½ cup almond milk

¼ cup almond butter

2 T local honey

1 T cinnamon

1 banana

Blend until smooth

Smoothies! Become a Smoothie Alchemist

Purify & Cleanse

2 cups chopped pineapple or canned

1/2 cup cottage cheese

1/4 cup milk

2 tsp. local honey

1/4 teaspoon vanilla

½ tsp. ground nutmeg

1/2 tsp. sea salt

2 cups crushed ice

Blend until smooth

Strong Start

½ cup cottage cheese

1 1/2 cup peach slices

½ cup unsweetened apple juice

1 tsp. local honey

Blend until smooth

Pineapple Princess

1 cup pineapple

1 mango

1 cup orange juice

1 cup Greek yogurt

Smoothies! Become a Smoothie Alchemist

Blend until smooth

Banana Beauty

1 banana

1 cup pineapple

1 cup coconut water

½ cup crushed ice

Blend until smooth

Inner Happiness

1 Banana

½ cup Peanut butter or Almond Butter

½ cup Skim milk

1 T local honey

½ cup crushed ice

Blend until smooth

Smoothies! Become a Smoothie Alchemist

Green Smoothies

Grace

6 romaine leaves, chopped

4 kale leaves, chopped

1/2 cup fresh parsley sprigs

1/2 cup chopped pineapple

1/2 cup chopped mango

1 inch fresh ginger, peeled and chopped

Blend until smooth

Wisdom Warrior

1 avocado

1 cup no-sugar-added pear nectar

2 kale leaves

1/2 teaspoon vanilla extract

1 cup crushed ice

Blend until smooth

Breath of Life

1 avocado

1/2 cup silken tofu drained

1 cup pear juice

2 T local honey

Smoothies! Become a Smoothie Alchemist

1/2 tsp. vanilla extract or stevia

2 cups crushed ice

Blend until smooth

Nirvana

1 ¼ cup coconut water

½ avocado

2 T walnuts

1 lime squeeze the juice

1 cup frozen mango

Blend until smooth

Well-being

2 bananas

1 cup Swiss chard leaves, stems removed

1 cup kale

1 apple

1/2 cup almond milk

Blend until smooth

Healthy Comfort

2 cups honeydew melon

1 cup almond milk

Smoothies! Become a Smoothie Alchemist

1 T local honey

Blend until smooth

Being in Balance

1 avocado

1 cup honeydew melon chunks

1 cup soy milk

½ cup unsweetened apple juice

1 tsp. local honey

Blend until smooth

Bliss

1 banana

½ cup frozen strawberries

1/2 cup frozen blueberries

1 peach

1 cup spinach

½ cup almond milk

½ Greek yogurt

2 tsp. local honey

1/2 cup crushed ice

Blend until smooth

Smoothies! Become a Smoothie Alchemist

Attitude Adjustment

1 1/2 cups green tea

1/3 cup almonds

1/4 cup honey

1 cup crushed ice

Blend until smooth

Pure Happiness

2 cups spinach

1 chopped peeled apple

1/2 cup silken tofu

¼ cup soy milk

¼ cup orange juice

1 T wheat germ

1 T local honey

1 T lemon juice

1 cup crushed ice

Blend until smooth

Calming Practice

1 cup kale

½ cucumber

1 apple, chopped

Smoothies! Become a Smoothie Alchemist

½ cup green grapes

1 orange

1 cup Romaine lettuce

¼ cup parsley

1 cup apple juice

½ cup crushed ice

Blend until smooth

Strawberry on a Mission

1 banana

1 cup strawberries

1 cup spinach, kale, or micro greens

6 fresh mint leaves

A little honey, maple syrup, or stevia to sweeten (optional)

1 cup filtered water

Blend until smooth

Chill Out

1 banana

1 cup seedless grapes

1 cup vanilla yogurt

1 apple, peeled, cored and cut into chunks

1-1/2 cups fresh spinach leaves

Smoothies! Become a Smoothie Alchemist

1/2 ripe avocado

½ cup crushed ice

Blend until smooth

Leadership

1/3 cup fresh mint

1 seeded jalapeno pepper

2 1/2 T. local honey

Pinch of sea salt

2 cups plain Greek yogurt

1 cup crushed ice

Blend until smooth

Top with toasted cumin seeds and cilantro

Forever Healthy

1/2 granny smith apple

1/2 cucumber

1 celery stalk, chopped

12 oz. green tea, brewed with 2 teabags

1 T fresh mint leaves

1/2 cup broccoli sprouts

1/2 cup watercress

½ cup crushed ice

Smoothies! Become a Smoothie Alchemist

Blend until smooth

Feel Good

1 large kale leaf, torn into pieces

1/2 cup coconut milk

1 cup apple juice

2 cups spinach

1 cup frozen mixed berries

½ cucumber

Blend until smooth

Green Conscience

½ cup parsley

1 cup pineapple

1 cucumber

½ cup crushed ice

Blend until smooth

Peace of Mind

1 1/4 cups almond milk

1/2 cup coconut water

2 leaves kale

1/2 avocado

Smoothies! Become a Smoothie Alchemist

1 mango, chopped

1/2 cup crushed ice

Blend until smooth

Honest Goodness

1/2 tsp. kelp

1 tsp. local honey

¼ cup pumpkin seeds

1 banana

1 orange

1 plum

1 peach

5 leaves chard

1 cup orange juice

½ cup crushed ice

Blend until smooth

Devotion to Health

1 apple

2 scoops wheat grass powder

2 cups spinach

1 cup green tea

6 oz. soy milk

Smoothies! Become a Smoothie Alchemist

1 cup ice cubes

Blend until smooth

Food is Life

½ cucumber

2 stalks celery, quartered

1 cup grapes any color

Coconut milk

1 grapefruit

Blend until smooth

You Renewed

1 cup kale

1 cup frozen cube mango

2 medium ribs celery, (chop into small pieces)

1 cup orange juice

¼ cup flat-leaf parsley

¼ cup fresh mint

Blend until smooth

Perfect Health

1 and 1/2 cups filtered water

1 banana

Smoothies! Become a Smoothie Alchemist

1 cup spinach

1 T spirulina powder

1 T cacao powder or nibs

¼ tsp. Ground cinnamon

¼ tsp. sea salt

1 T local honey

Blend until smooth

New Beginnings

3 cups kale

1/2 cup frozen blueberries

1/2 cup red frozen cranberries

1 banana

1/2 avocado

1/4 cup plain Greek yogurt

½ cup coconut milk

1/4 wedge of lemon, juice only

1/2 cup filtered water

Blend until smooth

Elixir of Life

1 cup unsweetened almond milk

1 cup packed chopped kale

Smoothies! Become a Smoothie Alchemist

1/2 cup pineapple juice

1/2 cup diced pineapple

1 banana

Blend until smooth

Centered

3 cups frozen white grapes

2 packed cups baby spinach

1 1/2 cups strong brewed green tea, cooled

1 avocado

2 tsp. honey

Blend until smooth

Human Nutrition

1 small cucumber

2 ripe kiwis

1 cup ginger-flavored kombucha

1/2 cup low-fat plain Greek yogurt

2 T cilantro leaves

½ cup crushed ice

Blend until smooth

Smoothies! Become a Smoothie Alchemist

Supreme Quality

1 1/2 cups hemp milk

1 banana

1-2 cups kale

1 T chia, flax, or hemp seeds

1 T coconut oil

¼ tsp. ground cinnamon

1 T local honey

Blend until smooth

Smoothies! Become a Smoothie Alchemist

Blue/Purple Smoothies

Good for the Soul

2 bananas

2/3 cup mango slices

1 12 ounce can grape juice, chilled

1 cup Greek yogurt

1 T local honey

Blend until smooth

2 tablespoons ground pistachio nuts

Fountain of Youth

1/2 cup frozen blueberries

1/2 cup frozen strawberries

1/2 cup chilled green tea

3/4 cup plain Greek yogurt

2 T ground flaxseed

Blend until smooth

Healthy Lifestyle

5 plums, quartered, pitted

1/2 cup buttermilk

1 cup vanilla frozen yogurt

Blend until smooth

Smoothies! Become a Smoothie Alchemist

Real Nourishment

1 cup frozen blackberries

1/2 cup frozen raspberries

1 cup vanilla yogurt

1 T local honey

Blend until smooth

Eat Smart

1 banana

1 cup blueberries

1/2 cup unsweetened coconut milk

1 T honey

1 T lime juice

1/4 teaspoon almond extract

½ cup crushed ice

Blend until smooth

Transformation Triple Berry

1 cup Greek vanilla yogurt

1 cup blackberries

1 cup strawberries

1 cup raspberries

Smoothies! Become a Smoothie Alchemist

1 cup almond milk

½ cup crushed ice

Blend until smooth

Fresh Finds

1 banana

1/2 cup blueberries

½ cup strawberries

½ cup raspberries

1/4 cup rolled oats

2 T chia seeds

1 1/2 cups almond milk

Blend until smooth

True Clarity

1 ripe banana

1 1/2 cups frozen blueberries

1 T lemon juice

3 T almond butter

2 T ground flaxseed

3 dates pitted

2 cups filtered water

Blend until smooth

Smoothies! Become a Smoothie Alchemist

Light of Awareness

1 1/2 cups frozen blackberries

1/2 cup low-fat plain yogurt

1/2 cup low-fat buttermilk

1 T honey

1/8 tsp. ground cinnamon

Blend until smooth

Rejuvenation

1 banana

1 cup low-fat Greek yogurt

1/3 cup seedless grapes

1/3 cup frozen blueberries

2 T frozen orange juice concentrate

Blend until smooth

The Inside Project

1/2 cup mango

1/2 cup blueberries

1/2 cup pineapple cubes

1 cup coconut water

Blend until smooth

Smoothies! Become a Smoothie Alchemist

Top with 1/4 cup chopped pumpkin seeds

Life Extension

1 ¼ cups apple juice

2 cups blueberries, frozen

1 kiwifruit, remove skin

Blend until smooth

Rediscover

1 and 1/2 cups filtered water

1/2 avocado

1/2 cup blueberries

1 T coconut oil

1/2 tsp. turmeric

1/2 tsp. ginger

1 T local honey

Blend until smooth

Truth Serum

1 cup blueberry juice

2 cups strawberries

1 cup Greek yogurt

2 T local honey

Smoothies! Become a Smoothie Alchemist

½ tsp. vanilla

Blend until smooth

Growth

¼ cup strawberries

¼ cup blueberries

¼ cup cherries

¼ cup raspberries

1 cup almond milk

1 tsp. chia seed

1 T agave nectar

Blend until smooth

Antioxidant Angel

2 cups mixed frozen berries

1 cup unsweetened pomegranate juice

1 cup water

Blend until smooth

Success

½ cup blueberries

½ cup pitted cherries

½ cup strawberries

Smoothies! Become a Smoothie Alchemist

1/2 avocado, peeled and pitted

2 tsp. wheat germ

2 tsp. ground flaxseed

1 cup almond or rice milk

Blend until smooth

I Love You

2 oranges, peel and pith removed, cut into chunks

1 cup frozen blueberries

1 cup frozen raspberries

1 T honey

Blend until smooth

Total Health

1 cup Greek yogurt

1 cup blueberries

1 banana

3 tsp. chia seeds

½ cup strawberries

1 cup orange Juice

Blend until smooth

Smoothies! Become a Smoothie Alchemist

The Athlete Within

1 cup blueberries

¾ cup beet juice

¾ cup pomegranate juice

1 T local honey

1 cup crushed ice

Blend until smooth

Eat Clean

1/2 cup blueberries, picked over and rinsed

1/2 cup low-fat vanilla yogurt

1/2 cup skim milk

2 T local honey

½ cup crushed ice

Blend until smooth

Eastern Delight

3 cups blackberries

1 cup plain low-fat yogurt

1 cup low-fat buttermilk

3 T local honey

½ tsp. ground cardamom

Blend until smooth

Smoothies! Become a Smoothie Alchemist

Rainbow of Health

1 ripe banana

1 cup frozen blueberries

1 cup plain Greek yogurt

Blend until smooth

Sun Warrior

1 banana

¼ cup fresh or frozen blueberries

¼ cup sliced fresh or frozen strawberries

¾ cup vanilla soymilk or milk

½ cup pomegranate juice, grape juice, or cranberry juice

½ cup vanilla frozen yogurt

Blend until smooth

Feel-Good

2 cups fresh baby spinach

1 cup blueberries

1 banana

½ cup vanilla yogurt

¼ cup chopped fresh pineapple

¼ cup frozen dark sweet cherries

¼ cup orange juice

Smoothies! Become a Smoothie Alchemist

Blend until smooth

It's Grape 2 B Alive

2 cups seedless red grapes

1 cup Concord grape juice

1 1/2 cups crushed ice

Blend until smooth

Tree of Life

1 1/2 cups frozen blueberries

1 chopped pear

1 1/2 cups each maple yogurt

1 cup crushed ice

Blend until smooth

Healthful Habits

2 navel oranges

1 cup frozen raspberries

1 cup frozen blueberries

1 kiwi

1 cup vanilla frozen yogurt

Blend until smooth

Smoothies! Become a Smoothie Alchemist

Indigo Goodness

1 cup berry yogurt

1 cup strawberries

1 cup raspberries

1 cup blueberries

1 cup almond or cashew milk

½ cup crushed ice

Blend until smooth

Drinking Wisdom

2 cups blueberries

1 cup low fat vanilla yogurt

6 ounces milk (any type)

1 cup pineapple juice

3 T local honey

Blend until smooth

Award Winning Smoothie

1 cup blueberries

1 cup Greek yogurt

1 cup Rice or any type milk

1 banana

½ cup crushed ice

Smoothies! Become a Smoothie Alchemist

Blend until smooth

A Feel Good Smoothie

1 cup blueberries

1 cup Greek yogurt

½ cup of fresh juice

1 banana

Handful of spinach

2 tablespoons of chocolate (pieces or powder)

Blend until smooth

Brown Smoothies

Comfort Smoothie

1 banana

3/4 cup kale

3/4 cup almond milk

3/4 T almond butter

1/8 tsp. cinnamon

1/8 tsp. nutmeg

1/8 tsp. ground ginger

Blend until smooth

Life-Centered

3 large chard leaves

1 banana

1 cup strawberries

1 cup raspberries

2 T sunflower seeds

1 T spirulina

1 cup orange juice

½ cup crushed ice

Blend until smooth

Smoothies! Become a Smoothie Alchemist

Pride

1 cup almond milk

½ cup reduced fat ricotta cheese

2 T hemp seeds

4 T maple syrup

1 cup frozen pitted dark cherries

Blend until smooth

Indulgence

1 T cacao powder

¼ cup Peanut butter

1 cup almond milk

12 peanuts

1 T local honey

½ cup crushed ice

Blend until smooth

Renaissance

1/2 cup coffee chilled

1/2 cup milk

3 T cashews

1 T coconut oil

1 T cacao powder

Smoothies! Become a Smoothie Alchemist

½ tsp. ground cinnamon

1/4 tsp. vanilla extract or stevia

¼ tsp. sea salt

1 T local honey

Blend until smooth

Think Clearly

1/3 cup almond milk

2 tsp. hemp seed

1 tsp. chia seed

1 T peanut butter

2 T rolled oats

Blend until smooth

Mocha Love

1 cup fat-free milk

1 banana

1 T local honey

1 T cacao powder

2 tsp. instant coffee crystals

½ tsp. vanilla

1 cup small ice cubes or crushed ice

Blend until smooth

Smoothies! Become a Smoothie Alchemist

Earth

1 cup soy milk

1 banana frozen

1 scoop chocolate whey protein

1 T peanut butter

1 cup frozen strawberries

Blend until smooth

Mother Earth

½ cup blueberries

½ cup strawberries

½ cup pineapple

1 cup baby spinach

1 banana

1 cup yogurt

2 carrots with the green top

1 oz. condensed cherry juice

12 raw almonds

1 tsp. cacao powder

1 cup almond milk

Blend until smooth

Smoothies! Become a Smoothie Alchemist

Feed Your Brain

1 cup almond milk

1 banana

2 T peanut butter

1 tsp. cinnamon

1 scoop whey protein powder

1 tsp. chia seeds

Blend until smooth

Eternal Health

1 banana

1 T peanut butter

1/2 cup frozen berries

1 cup unsweetened almond milk

2 kale leaves

1 scoop protein powder

Blend until smooth

Live!

2 cup frozen chocolate yogurt

½ cup milk (any type)

4 tablespoons peanut butter

Blend until smooth

Smoothies! Become a Smoothie Alchemist

Inspiration

1 cup low-fat buttermilk

2 bananas

11 dried pitted dates soak for several hours

1 tsp. local honey

Pinch of salt

½ cup crushed ice

Blend until smooth

Connection

2 1/2 pears

1 3/4 cups skim milk

1 cup low-fat buttermilk

2/3 cup rolled oats

2 T maple syrup

2 T almond butter

1 1/4 tsp. finely grated fresh ginger

1/8 tsp. ground cinnamon

1 tsp. sea salt

1/3 cup ice cubes

Blend until smooth

Smoothies! Become a Smoothie Alchemist

Revitalize

1/4 cup almond butter

2 cardamom pods or 1 teaspoon ground cardamom

1 1/2 cups filtered water

1 cup frozen peaches

1 to 2 tsp. agave syrup

1/2 cup crushed ice

Blend until smooth

Balanced Body

2 frozen bananas

3/4 cup chopped pitted dates

1 lime juice and zest

1 1/2 cups soy milk

½ cup crushed ice

Blend until smooth

Inner Support

1 banana

2 dates pitted, soak several hours

1 cup milk (any type)

1 T wheat germ

4 leaves of romaine lettuce

Smoothies! Become a Smoothie Alchemist

1 T cacao powder

½ cup crushed ice

Blend until smooth

Awaken!

1/2 cup chilled espresso or strong coffee

1/2 cup milk or almond milk

1 T. xylitol

1/4 tsp. ground cinnamon

1/8 tsp. almond extract

1 cup crushed ice

Blend until smooth

Renewed

1/2 cup chilled espresso or strong coffee

1/4 cup sweetened condensed milk

1 1/2 cups crushed ice

Blend until smooth

Top with dark chocolate shavings

Stay Well

1 frozen banana

1 cup soy milk

Smoothies! Become a Smoothie Alchemist

¼ cup peanut butter

¼ cup wheat germ

2 T seedless strawberry jelly

Blend until smooth

Cup of Intelligence

1 apple

3 T peanut butter

2 T flax seeds

1 1/2 cups soy milk

1 cup crushed ice

1 T local honey

Blend until smooth

Compassion

1 banana

1 cup vanilla Greek yogurt

1/2 cup peanut butter

1/3 cup milk (any type)

2 T malted milk powder

1/2 tsp. cacao powder

1 tsp. sea salt

1 cup crushed ice

Smoothies! Become a Smoothie Alchemist

Blend until smooth

Empowerment

1 cup frozen chocolate yogurt

1/4 cup cacao nibs

1/2 cup almond milk

Blend until smooth

Inner Strength and Beauty

1 cup almond milk

¼ cup goji berries

Handful of spinach or kale leaves

3 T cacao nibs

½ cup crushed ice

Blend until smooth

Focus

2 tsp. cacao powder

3 tsp. local honey

1 cup skim milk

1 cup vanilla frozen yogurt

Blend until smooth

Now it's your turn to become a Smoothie Alchemist.

Choose to live well,

Kimberly Wechsler

www.ingramcontent.com/pod-product-compliance
Lightning Source LLC
Chambersburg PA
CBHW061454040426
42450CB00007B/1354